MIX
Papier aus verantwortungsvollen Quellen
Paper from responsible sources
FSC® C105338

Bernt-Dieter Huismans
Wolfgang Klemann
Stephan Heyl

Prolonged antibiotic therapy in PCR confirmed persistent Lyme disease

Anchor Compact

Huismans, Bernt-Dieter, Klemann, Wolfgang, Heyl, Stephan: Prolonged antibiotic therapy in PCR confirmed persistent Lyme disease, Hamburg, Anchor Academic Publishing 2014

Original title of the thesis: Prolonged antibiotic therapy in PCR confirmed persistent Lyme disease

Buch-ISBN: 978-3-95489-241-9
PDF-eBook-ISBN: 978-3-95489-741-4
Druck/Herstellung: Anchor Academic Publishing, Hamburg, 2014

Bibliografische Information der Deutschen Nationalbibliothek:
Die Deutsche Nationalbibliothek verzeichnet diese Publikation in der Deutschen Nationalbibliografie; detaillierte bibliografische Daten sind im Internet über http://dnb.d-nb.de abrufbar

Bibliographical Information of the German National Library:
The German National Library lists this publication in the German National Bibliography. Detailed bibliographic data can be found at: http://dnb.d-nb.de

All rights reserved. This publication may not be reproduced, stored in a retrieval system or transmitted, in any form or by any means, electronic, mechanical, photocopying, recording or otherwise, without the prior permission of the publishers.

Das Werk einschließlich aller seiner Teile ist urheberrechtlich geschützt. Jede Verwertung außerhalb der Grenzen des Urheberrechtsgesetzes ist ohne Zustimmung des Verlages unzulässig und strafbar. Dies gilt insbesondere für Vervielfältigungen, Übersetzungen, Mikroverfilmungen und die Einspeicherung und Bearbeitung in elektronischen Systemen.

Die Wiedergabe von Gebrauchsnamen, Handelsnamen, Warenbezeichnungen usw. in diesem Werk berechtigt auch ohne besondere Kennzeichnung nicht zu der Annahme, dass solche Namen im Sinne der Warenzeichen- und Markenschutz-Gesetzgebung als frei zu betrachten wären und daher von jedermann benutzt werden dürften.

Die Informationen in diesem Werk wurden mit Sorgfalt erarbeitet. Dennoch können Fehler nicht vollständig ausgeschlossen werden und die Diplomica Verlag GmbH, die Autoren oder Übersetzer übernehmen keine juristische Verantwortung oder irgendeine Haftung für evtl. verbliebene fehlerhafte Angaben und deren Folgen.

Alle Rechte vorbehalten

© Anchor Academic Publishing, ein Imprint der Diplomica® Verlag GmbH
http://www.diplom.de, Hamburg 2014
Printed in Germany

Abstract: We examined a sample of 90 individuals that had previously received a course of appropriate antibiotics for Lyme disease without experiencing full resolution of their symptoms and had evidence of persistent infection documented by PCR analysis.

Mean duration of symptoms was 9.5 years (range 1 - 40 years). The treatment was adapted to the individual case according to clinical response. Long term antibiotic therapy was initiated and patients were treated continuously for at least 6 months, in some cases several years of intermittent therapy was administered. About 38.8% of the patients experienced full remission of symptoms while about 56.7% reported a significant improvement, 5.6% of patients were deemed refractory to therapy. Therapeutic modalities are discussed in detail.

Key words: persistent Lyme disease, Borrelia PCR, long term antibiotic treatment, lyme serology, Borrelia DNA

Key issues:
- All study patients were Borrelia- DNA positive
- Commonly reported symptoms included fatigue, muscular- skeletal and neuro-psychiatric complaints
- Only about 42% of patients had a history of an erythema migrans
- Serologic testing is fairly insensitive in late disseminated lyme disease
- Antibiotic treatment must be tailored to the individual clinical response in late disseminated lyme disease
- The majority of patients benefited from long term antibiotic treatment
- Recurrence of symptoms was common during treatment
- Long term antibiotic therapy was generally well tolerated

Table of Content

Introduction 7
Patients 9
Detection of borrelial DNA in skin biopsies 13
Therapeutic rationale 14
Antibiotic therapy 14
    Tetracyclines 14
    Beta- lactam antibiotics 15
    Macrolides 15
    Nitroimidazoles 16
    Lysosomotropic agents 16
    Other antibiotics 16
Treatment strategies 18
Rationale for combination therapy 18
Treatment course 19
Treatment results 20
Summary and discussion 22
    Expert commentary and five- year view 24
Articles 26

Introduction

Lyme disease was first described as an independent entity by Allen C. Steere et. al. [1] in 1977. Since then we have learned that this complex illness is the result of an infectious process, that not only affects the skin and joints but can potentially disseminate systemically. Although 30 years have passed since the discovery of the disease, the available data on therapy still has to be considered sparse. In a review article published in 2006 D. Hassler summarized the available data on the treatment of lyme disease and commented on the paucity of evidence [2]. Only a few controlled studies and some in vitro observations are available. Nevertheless certain standards have been established and have made their way into treatment guidelines. Two currently available guidelines are widely accepted, one is published by the Infectious Diseases Society of America (IDSA) [3], the other by the International Lyme and Associated Diseases Society (ILADS) [4]. The two guidelines propose strikingly different approaches for the treatment of late stage Lyme disease.

Previous studies usually included patients that were diagnosed with Lyme borreliosis based on clinical and serologic findings most of which were in an early stage of the disease [5, 6]. These serological criteria were introduced primarily for epidemiologic purposes reasons and lack sensitivity [4, 7] for clinical use. It is doubtful whether results obtained from these studies can be generalized and applied to other cases of lyme disease. Articles that document cases diagnosed by detection of borrelial DNA have, to our knowledge, been limited to case reports and case series [8,9]. For this article we have gathered a large number of patients that were diagnosed with late stage lyme disease based on clinical and serological findings as well as direct evidence of the causative microorganism by using polymerase chain reaction (PCR). We provide long term follow up on the clinical course and treatment of these patients and evaluate the efficacy of prolonged courses (range 6-60 months) of antibiotics in these patients.

Patients

Patients sought medical attention between 1998 and 2007 because of persistent symptoms despite a presumably adequate course of antibiotics for Lyme disease. To be included in this analysis the patients had to have demonstrable *Borrelia* DNA (PCR method) in a skin sample in conjunction with the presence of clinical signs and symptoms consistent with Lyme disease.

Patient characteristics:
- *Borrelia* DNA detected in skin biopsies of all patients
- Despite adequate course of antibiotics in the past ongoing symptoms and signs most typical for Lyme Disease
- 36.66% (33/90) of patients were male, 63.33% (57/90) were female
- All age groups present, mean age 49, range 7- 88 years
- 42.22% (38/90) recalled skin rash consistent with erythema migrans
- Increased LFTs in 19% of patients
- Mean duration of illness 9.5 years (range 1-40 years) as shown in figure 1

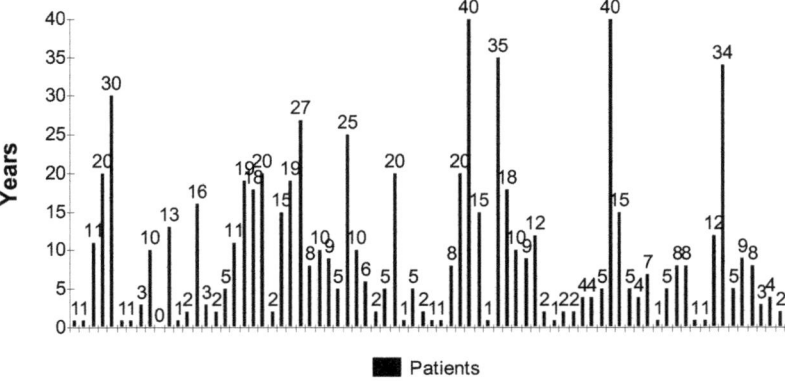

Figure 1: Duration in years from onset of symptoms until first administration of antibiotics (Only data from 76/90 patients was available)

The most commonly reported symptoms were fatigue, musculoskeletal and neuropsychiatric complaints (see figure 2). This observation is similar to that found in the current literature. [10, 11]. The severity of the symptoms ranged from relatively mild to disabling. Most patients had already seen many specialists about their persistent complaints.

To be included in the study the patients had to have skin manifestations, in most cases clinically diagnosed acrodermatitis chronica atrophicans or recurrent erythema migrans as a manifestation of disseminated disease.

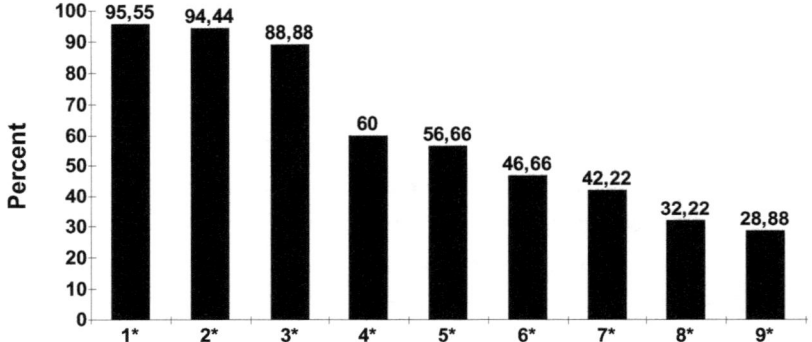

Figure 2: The frequency of clinical symptoms and findings. 1*. Neuropsychiatric, 2*. Musculo- skeletal 3*. Fatigue, 4*. Gastrointestinal [10], 5*. Eye manifestations, 6*. Cardiac, 7*. History of Erythema migrans 8*. Hypertension, 9*. Thyroid disease

Many of the patients had serologic evidence of co-infections (e.g. *Chlamydia spp.*, *Mycoplasma spp.*, *Yersinia enterocolitica* or *others*) or non- infectious comorbidities. We evaluated 42/ 90 patients for co-infections. 80.6% (25/31) were positive for *Chlamydia spp.*, 78.3 % (18/23) for *Mycoplasma spp.* and 77.8% for *Yersinia* (7/9). The seroprevalence of these infections was considerably higher among our sample than the seroprevalence reported among the general population [12, 13, 14]. The reasons for this surprising finding are unclear, although one could speculate that our patient sample was more prone to infection than the general population because of their persistent Lyme disease. Treatment was considered in cases of detectable IgM / IgA response. Coinfected patients tended to have more severe disease and often needed combination therapy.

Serologic testing by ELISA and Western blot was performed on all patients. Surprisingly, only 57% of patients had a positive Borrelia serology, even though all had PCR confirmed disease. The serologic findings of our sample are shown in figure 3. The IgG western blot exhibited the highest degree of sensitivity (58%). Only 43.52% (37/85) of patients had both a positive ELISA test and a positive Western blot, while in 10.85% (9/85) the positive ELISA result was not confirmed by the Western blot. In 24.70% (21/85) of cases the ELISA test remained negative despite a positive Western blot, even though, to be useful as a screening tool, the ELISA test should theoretically exhibit higher sensitivity. These results question the often recommended two- tiered testing approach [3, 4, 7], since some patients with a negative ELISA test will still have a strongly positive Western blot.

The lack of sensitivity of serologic testing for lyme disease has been described [8, 9, 15, 16] and commercially available kits are not standardized and produce dramatically different results in some cases.

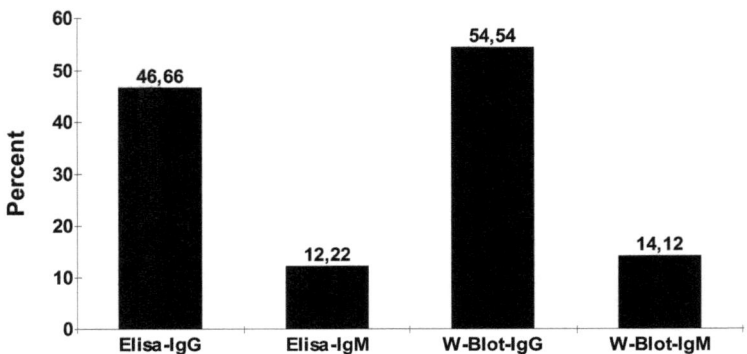

Figure 3: Positive serological findings in study patients

Detection of borrelial DNA in skin biopsies

Author of this section: ZeckLab, Labor für Klinische Diagnostik und Prüfung, Dr. Gabriele Liebisch/Prof. Dr. Arndt Liebisch

Skin biopsies were examined by nested PCR to ensure high specificity. The skin biopsy was cut into small pieces (0.5 mm) using a sterile scalpel blade and the DNA was purified using the QIAamp® DNA Mini Kit. Purification was done after incubation with proteinase K and elution of the DNA was performed using DNAse / RNAse free water. This DNA was employed as a template for the PCR reaction. The SL- primers [17] were used as outer primers for the first PCR run and the nested PCR MRL7/MRL11 [18] primer pair was used as inner primers for the second PCR run. Analysis was performed after the addition of SYBR®-Green and agarose gel electrophoresis by comparing the PCR product to a DNA molecular weight marker. Amplification was done in a Speed Cycler (Analytik Jena). For the first run using the outer primer pair 40 cycles were performed. Denaturation at 94°C for 4 s, annealing at 55°C for 4s and elongation at 72 °C for 25 s. At the end of the 40 cycles, another elongation step at 72 °C for 3 min was done. 3 µl of the PCR product of the first run were used as template DNA for the second run using the same durations and temperature conditions as for the first run.

Outer Primer Sequence

BBSL1   5'- AAT AGG TCT AAT AAT AGC CTT AAT AGC- 3'

BBSL2   5'- CTA GTG TTT TGC CAT CTT CTT TGA AAA -3'

Inner Primer Sequence

MRL7   5'- GTT TCA GTA GAT TTG CCT GG-3'

MRL11   5-' CCT TCA AGT ACT CCA GAT CC-3'

This PCR procedure allowed for the reproducible detection of several borrelial species (*B.burgdorferi* B31, *B. afzelii* and B.garinii) in skin biopsies. A study by Schnarr et al. demonstrated successful detection of borrelial DNA in synovial fluid using this procedure [19].

Therapeutic rationale

Since our patient sample was positive for borrelial DNA despite a previous course of antibiotics we considered ongoing infection to be the primary cause of the patients' persistent complaints. Our therapeutic goal was therefore the elimination of the causative organism, *B. burgdorferi* through antibiotic therapy.

In addition to antibiotic treatment of the patients lifestyle modifications were recommended. Those included the regular exercise, balanced diet, stress regulation, heat application and abstinence from drugs, nicotine and alcohol. Where indicated symptomatic treatment with NSAIDs, antidepressants and anticonvulsants was initiated.

Compliance with the recommended lifestyle changes was satisfactory, however, about 15% of patients continued to smoke or imbibe larger quantities of alcohol.

Antibiotic therapy

We used antibiotics whose efficacy was confirmed by clinical trials and in- vitro studies for the treatment of Lyme disease. The unique lifecycle and biology of B. burgdorferi were also taken into consideration when selecting suitable antibiotic agents [1, 2, 3, 4, 5, 6].

Tetracyclines

Initially, we usually started our patients on a tetracycline derivative because tetracyclines are also active against several co-infections and intracellular organisms. In more severe cases, IV Doxycycline was employed followed by oral doxycycline or tetracycline. Tetracycline may have advantages over doxycycline since, despite lower absorption rate from the GI tract, higher serum levels can be achieved since the total dose given is much higher (200mg total dose daily for doxycycline and 1500 mg total dose daily for tetracycline) and the amount of free drug available is higher with tetracycline [20].

Since it is very inconvenient to administer more than one dose of antibiotic intravenously in an ambulatory setting, doxycycline was mostly combined with tetracycline using the following dosages: IV doxycycline 200 mg / day (diluted in 100 ml of normal saline) and tetracycline 2x500 mg / day orally for at least 20 days. Depending on the patient's response this cycle could be repeated several times.
Based on pharmacokinetic considerations (higher lipophilicity and better penetration into the cerebrospinal fluid) we also used minocycline 2x100 mg /day with good success [21].

Beta- lactam antibiotics

Ceftriaxone was the preferred antibiotic from the beta- lactam family since this substance has been evaluated in several studies [22, 23]. It was prescribed using dosages from 2 to 4 g / day depending on the patient's weight. At first the infusions were administered on a daily basis for 21 days, followed by pulsed therapy on 3-4 days/week. Pulsed therapy was continued until sustained clinical benefit was evident.
In severe cases of refractory neuroborreliosis cefotaxime was administered in a dosage of 4g three times daily instead of ceftriaxone.

Macrolides

From the group of macrolides clarithromycine was prescribed predominantly. In more severe cases, intravenous application was preferred at least initially, followed by oral administration once improvement was seen. In case of an unsatisfactory response combination therapy using macrolids, hydroxychloroquine and/or tetracyclines was administered. The use of Clarithromycin in early disease is supported by a trial by Dattwyler et al. [24]. In late Lyme disease it is supported by an uncontrolled trial by Donta et al., which demonstrated good results using macrolides in combination with hydroxychloroquine [10]. In select cases dual inhibition of bacterial protein synthesis using a macrolide antibiotic and a tetracycline produced excellent results.

Nitroimidazoles

Out of concern for cystic Borrelia forms nitroimidazoles have been used in patients in whom other antibiotic regimens had failed [25, 26, 27]. Although the clinical relevance of cystic forms has been disputed [28], in our experience some patients benefit significantly from a 10 day course. The preferred agent was IV metronidazole 500mg twice daily, an additional 400mg tablet was given in the late evening. Combination therapy with doxycycline or a macrolide antibiotic is also a possibility in refractory cases.

Lysosomotropic agents

Lysosomotropic agents, mostly hydroxychloroquine [10] was also used in dosages from 200 to 400 mg / day mainly in combination with macrolide antibiotics, occasionally also with doxycycline. Intracellular bacteria are often held in an acidic vacuole, which renders certain antibiotics ineffective [29]. Lysosomotropic agents alkalize this vacuole, thereby increasing the antibiotic-effectiveness`. Hydroxychloroquine may additionally have some efficacy against cystic forms [30] and it's anti- inflammatory properties can be useful as well.

Other antibiotics

In case of co-infections or if the patient was unable to tolerate the preferred antibiotic regiments we switched the patients to second line therapies. This was necessary in about 14% of the patients.
In this group of other antibiotics are included:
- Imipenem (in patients unable to tolerate ceftriaxone) [31]
- Rifampin usually in combination with macrolides for the treatment of co-infections (e.g. *Chlamydia* [32])

- IM Penicillin G benzathine [33]
- Vancomycin [34] in cases of multiple allergies

Treatment strategies

Rather than treating our patients for an arbitrary amount of time, duration of treatment depended on the individual clinical response. As a consequence of this approach the total duration of treatment differed from patient to patient (range 6-60 months). In many cases, improvement was only seen after 5- 6 weeks of therapy and it usually took even more time to achieve improvement that was sustained when the antibiotic was withdrawn. We considered switching the patient to a different antibiotic when 4- 6 weeks had elapsed without improvement. If no improvement was seen after several cycles of antibiotics and/or combination therapy the treatment was classified as a failure.

Rationale for combination therapy

Several arguments favor combination therapy over treatment with a single agent:
- long term therapy is needed for sustained clinical improvement in many cases
- therapy with a single agent is often not sufficiently effective
- that many other pathogens (for example *H. pylori*, *M. tuberculosis* or *C. burnetii*) are only successfully treated with a combination of antibiotics

In the past three years we have used several combinations of antibiotics with good results [35, 36]. This was attempted particularly in those cases where therapy with a single agent was unsuccessful or in the presence of co-infections. In general, combination therapy was tolerated fairly well. Even though it is mentioned in the ILADS guidelines [4], not many studies on this subject are available at this point. More research and controlled trials are needed to assess the efficacy of combination therapy over monotherapy.

Treatment course

Often in the beginning of the therapy worsening of symptoms occurred. This may be the result of a Jarisch- Herxheimer like reaction caused by bacterial lysis and the secretion of pro-inflammatory cytokines [37]. This reaction was rarely severe and only isolated cases required short term treatment with a corticosteroid.

It was uncommon for patients to be symptom free after short (up to 4 weeks) courses of antibiotics. Usually many months passed until significant improvement occurred, and this time varied significantly from case to case. The longer the patient was ill before therapy was instated, the more aggressive therapy was needed to achieve sustained improvement in the patient's condition. This observation is unfortunately consistent with data from other reports [4, 20].

In general at least 6 months of treatment were necessary for sustained improvement and 3-5 years of intermittent therapy was often needed to achieve full remission.

During the antibiotic therapy we routinely checked the following parameters:

Every 8 to 14 days:
- blood pressure, CBC, GGT, ALT, serum creatinine

Every 2 to 4 weeks:
- focused physical exam

Every 3 months:
- ECG (particularly in patients taking macrolide antibiotics or hydroxychloroquine)
- during hydroxychloroquine treatment: fundoscopy

Treatment results

Full remission was defined as the complete resolution of the patients' Lyme associated symptoms and clinical findings for at least six months. This was observed in 37. 8 % of patients (see figure 4: treatment results). About 56. 8% of the patients reported a significant improvement during treatment, but eventually their symptoms recurred or new symptoms developed. These relapses could usually be treated by additional courses of antibiotic therapy. Using these measures these relapses occurred less commonly and decreased in severity but for the purpose of this article these patients were not considered to be in full remission. For about 5.4% of patients no improvement was seen after antibiotic therapy.

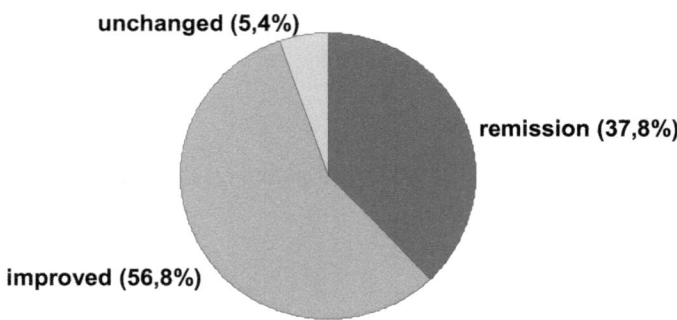

Figure 4: Treatment results

Serious treatment complications were extremely rare. About 8% of patients developed mild to moderate allergic reactions (usually allergic rashes) during the treatment, the antibiotic regime were changed in this case.
Adverse events were most commonly observed during treatment with ceftriaxone. Two patients had to undergo cholecystectomies because of gall stones associated with prolonged ceftriaxone therapy. Ceftriaxone induced pseudolithiasis is a fairly common complication, fortunately the condition seems to be reversible after stopping the drug [38]. Most of the adverse events were mild in nature, two severe

Herxheimer like reactions were observed which had to be treated with corticosteroids and antihistamines.

One case of urinary retention was observed in a patient with a history of Parkinson's disease who was treated with amantadine.

Summary and discussion

Currently no reliable standards for the treatment of persistent Lyme disease and relevant co-infections [3, 4] have been established and no antibiotic regimen has been shown to yield clinically superior outcomes [38].

In this study we evaluated the effects of longer treatment cycles in individuals that had been previously been treated unsuccessfully for several weeks. Despite previous treatment *Borrelia* DNA was demonstrable in skin biopsies of those patients, which was unlikely to be due to reinfection. Our approach used an individually adapted treatment strategy with long term antibiotic therapy of 6 to 60 months duration that was guided by clinical improvement. Patients who failed to improve were evaluated for the presence of co-infections. This approach is similar to the one outlined in the ILADS guidelines [4]. Furthermore the well described anti- inflammatory effects of certain antibiotics may have had some positive effect in some cases [39, 40], although these effects are unlikely to be of permanent or even prolonged duration.

Using this strategy about 37.8% (34/90) of the patients experienced a complete remission of their symptoms while about 56.7% (51/90) reported feeling significantly improved. Solely 5.6% of the patients were deemed refractory to antibtiotic therapy. These observations challenge the view that long term therapy for disseminated lyme disease is ineffective [28, 41] and provide further support that long term antibiotic therapy is worthwhile [20, 4, 10, 11]. More research regarding the optimal treatment regimen and duration is needed.

It is not clear why some patients need more intensive antibiotic therapy than others. Co-infections, the unique biology of *Borrelia burgdorferi*, it's ability to evade the immune response of the host and immunological factors probably play a role. In his review article RB Stricker summarizes the complex microbiology of *B. burgdorferi* that may lead to therapeutic failure [35]. It has recently been demonstrated that a four week course of ceftriaxone not only fails to eradicate B. burgdorferi infection in mice but the remaining spirochetes are still infectious [42]. Moreover, treatment of antibiotically treated, Lyme infected mice with tumor necrosis factor α blocking agents can reactivate latent infection [43].

Our patient sample contained 63, 3% (57/90) women, and in some families multiple family members were affected. This suggests that hormonal and genetic factors may play a role in the pathogenesis of persistent Lyme disease and these factors may even determine individual susceptibility [43, 45, 20]. Additional research in this area to find out why some patients with acute Lyme borreliosis are easily treatable while some go on to develop chronic sequelae is needed.

In addition to antibiotic therapy certain lifestyle modifications are recommended to maximize the treatment effect. Avoidance of stressful activities, alcohol, nicotine and other recreational drugs is essential. A graded physical exercise program helps the patients who are often chronically debilitated regain their strength. On certain occasions symptomatic treatment for pain and neuropsychiatric symptoms is indicated in order to normalize the patients' day to day activities.

This case series underscores the need for more randomized controlled trials of longer courses of antibiotics in chronic Lyme disease. The present work should only be understood as a pilot study since the results were obtained retrospectively from patients in a medical private practice. Klempner et al. published a study in 2001 which compared 30 days of IV ceftriaxone therapy followed by 60 days of oral doxycycline with placebo [41]. While considerable impairment in the quality of life of the study participants was seen, no treatment effect was observed. This study has been subject to controversial discussion: one side maintains that we should abandon long term antibiotic therapy for persistent Lyme disease altogether, while the other side notes significant flaws in the study's design [35, 46, 47, 48]. These flaws concern mainly the inclusion criteria, the antibiotic regimen, treatment duration and the scales used to measure improvement in the patient's condition. While we consider the study to be important, it does not demonstrate that long term antibiotic therapy regardless of therapeutic regimen is ineffective, especially since PCR positive patients were specifically excluded. Our case series shows that patients with PCR proven persistent Lyme borreliosis may benefit greatly from prolonged therapy.

In 2008 another placebo controlled treatment study was published by B. Fallon et al [11]. The study included patients that were seropositive, had received previous antibiotic treatment and had objectifiable cognitive deficits. The participants were randomized to 10 weeks of IV ceftriaxone or IV placebo. At the end of the treatment period, improvement was seen across all domains, however, this improvement was not sustained after the antibiotic was discontinued. This result is similar to what we have experienced in clinical practice: insufficiently treated patients will relapse after the antibiotic has been withdrawn. Often, these patients can be successfully treated by a longer course of antibiotics.

Dealing with patients that suffer from long- term complaints attributable to Lyme borreliosis can be difficult. While there is evidence that a proportion of patients is still symptomatic after presumably adequate antibiotic therapy [49] there is, even among experts, considerable dissent concerning the etiology, pathogenesis and optimal therapy for these patients [35, 50, 53]. Therefore a lot of responsibility rests with the individual physician to make informed treatment decisions [36]. It has been our experience that long term antibiotic treatment is worth trying in persistent Lyme disease since it can be surprisingly effective in persistent Lyme disease, even in cases with long standing symptoms. From this clinical viewpoint we stipulate that persistent Lyme disease is due to ongoing infection rather than the result of an as yet ill- defined post-infectious / autoimmune process.

Expert commentary and five- year view

To further our understanding of this complex illness more research into the molecular mechanisms of persistence of *Borrelia* is needed. More studies on the effect co-infections have on the course of the disease are necessary as well. Clinically, Anaplasma, Mycoplasma, Babesia and Bartonella coinfection can be difficult to distinguish from classic Lyme borreliosis [51, 52].
Considering the clinical and microbiological complexity of Lyme disease clinicians and researchers need to keep an open mind and should not be afraid to explore new ways of looking at and dealing with Borrelia burgdorferi. We should also be careful about applying diagnostic criteria that were designed for research to real clinical patients, as the disease process is so variable that some patients may then be denied appropriate care. Only then will we be able to relieve the suffering caused by this illness and deal with the enormous economic burden it represents.

Articles

[1] Steere AC, Malawista SE, Snydman DR, et al (1977). "Lyme arthritis: an epidemic of oligoarticular arthritis in children and adults in three connecticut communities". *Arthritis Rheum.* 20 (1): 7–17 (1977).

[2] Hassler D, Phasengerechte Therapie der Lyme-Borreliose. *Chemother J* 15, 106-111 (2006)

[3] Wormser GP, Nadelman RB, Dattwyler RJ, et al. "Practice guidelines for the treatment of Lyme disease. The Infectious Diseases Society of America" *Clin Infect Dis* 31 (Suppl 1): 1-14 (2000).

[4] Cameron D, Gaito A, Narris N, et. al. ILADS Working Group "Evidence-based guidelines for the management of Lyme disease". *Expert Rev Anti Infect Ther* 2 (1 Suppl): S1-13 (2004).

[5] Dattwyler RJ, Volkman DJ, Conaty SM, Platkin SP, et al. Amoxycillin plus probenecid versus doxycycline for treatment of erythema migrans borreliosis. *Lancet*; 336:1404–6 (1990).

[6] Steere AC, Hutchinson GJ, Rahn DW, Sigal LH, et al. Treatment of the early manifestations of Lyme disease. *Ann Intern Med.* 99: 22–6 (1983)

[7] Stricker RB, Lautin A, Burrascano JJ. Lyme disease: point/counterpoint. *Expert Rev Anti Infect Ther.* 3(2), 155-65, (2005)

[8] Oksi J, Uksila J, Marjamäki M, Nikoskelainen J, Viljanen MK Antibodies against whole sonicated Borrelia burgdorferi spirochetes, 41-kilodalton flagellin, and P39 protein in patients with PCR- or culture-proven late Lyme borreliosis. *J Clin Microbiol.* 33(9):2260-4 (1995).

[9] Chmielewski T, Fiett J, Gniadkowski M, Tylewska-Wierzbanowska S. Improvement in the laboratory recognition of lyme borreliosis with the combination of culture and PCR methods. *Mol Diagn.* 7(3-4):155-62 (2003).

[10] Donta ST, Macrolide therapy of chronic Lyme Disease. *Med Sci Monit.* 9(11) 136-142 (2003)

[11] Fallon BA, Keilp JG, Corbera KM et al. A randomized, placebo-controlled trial of repeated IV antibiotic therapy for Lyme encephalopathy. *Neurology* 70(13):992-1003 (2008)

[12] Liu FC, Chen PY, Huang FL, Tsai CR, Lee CY, Lin CF. Do Serological Tests Provide Adequate Rapid Diagnosis of Mycoplasma pneumoniae Infection? *Jpn J Infect Dis.* 61(5):397-9 (2008).

[13] Tomaso H, Mooseder G, Dahouk SA, et al. Seroprevalence of anti-Yersinia antibodies in healthy Austrians. *Eur J Epidemiol.* 21(1):77-81 (2006).

[14] Paldanius M, Bloigu A, Leinonen M, Saikku P. Measurement of Chlamydia pneumoniae-specific immunoglobulin A (IgA) antibodies by the microimmunofluorescence (MIF) method: comparison of seven fluorescein-labeled anti-human IgA conjugates in an in-house MIF test using one commercial MIF and one enzyme immunoassay kit. *Clin Diagn Lab Immunol.* 10(1):8-12 (2003).

[15] Coulter P, Lema C, Flayhart D et al. Two-year evaluation of Borrelia burgdorferi culture and supplemental tests for definitive diagnosis of Lyme disease. *J Clin Microbiol.* 43(10):5080-4 (2005) Erratum in: *J Clin Microbiol.* 45(1):277 (2007).

[16] Mouritsen CL, Wittwer CT, Litwin CM et al. Polymerase chain reaction detection of Lyme disease: correlation with clinical manifestations and serologic responses. *Am J Clin Pathol.* 105(5):647-54 (1996).

[17] Demaerschalck I, Ben Messaoud A, De Kesel M et al. Simultaneous presence of different Borrelia burgdorferi genospecies in biological fluids of Lyme disease patients. *J Clin Microbiol.* 33(3):602-8 (1995).

[18] Liebling MR, Nishio MJ, Rodriguez A, Sigal LH, Jin T, Louie JS. The polymerase chain reaction for the detection of Borrelia burgdorferi in human body fluids. *Arthritis Rheum.* 36(5):665-75 (1993).

[19] Schnarr S, Jürgens- Saathoff B, Liebisch G et al. Optimierung einer PCR zum Nachweis von Borrelia burgdorferi sensu lato in Synovialflüssigkeit *Z. Rheumatol.* 57, 37 (1998)

[20] Donta ST, Tetracycline Therapy for Chronic Lyme Disease. *Clin Infect Dis* 1, 52-56 (1997)

[21] Liegner KB, Minocycline in Lyme disease. *J. Am. Acad. Dermatol.* 26, 263-264 (1992)

[22] Dattwyler RJ, Wormser GP, Rush TJ, et al. A comparison of two treatment regimens of ceftriaxone in late Lyme disease. *Wien Klin Wochenschr.* 117(11-12):393-7 (2005).

[23] Dattwyler RJ, Halperin JJ, Volkman DJ, Luft BJ. Treatment of late Lyme borreliosis--randomised comparison of ceftriaxone and penicillin. *Lancet* 1(8596):1191-4 (1988).

[24] Dattwyler RJ, Grunwaldt E, Luft BJ. Clarithromycin in treatment of early Lyme disease: a pilot study. *Antimicrob Agents Chemother.* 40(2):468-9 (1996).

[25] Brorson O, Brorson SH. An in vitro study of the susceptibility of mobile and cystic forms of Borrelia burgdorferi to metronidazole. *APMIS.* 107(6):566-76 (1999).

[26] Brorson O, Brorson SH. An in vitro study of the susceptibility of mobile and cystic forms of Borrelia burgdorferi to tinidazole. *Int Microbiol.* 7(2):139-42 (2004).

[27] Alban PS, Johnson PW, Nelson DR. Serum-starvation-induced changes in protein synthesis and morphology of Borrelia burgdorferi. *Microbiology* 146:119-127 (2000).

[28] Feder H, Johnson B, Shapiro E et al. A Critical Appraisal of „Chronic Lyme Disease". *N. Engl. J. Med.* 357(14), 1422-1430 (2007), Correction 358 (10) 1084 (2008)

[29] Rolain JM, Colson P, Raoult D. Recycling of chloroquine and its hydroxyl analogue to face bacterial, fungal and viral infections in the 21st century. *Int J Antimicrob Agents.* 30(4):297-308 (2007)

[30] Brorson O, Brorson SH, An in vitro study ot the susceptibility of mobile and cystic forms of Borrelia burgdorferi to hydroxichloroquine. *Int Microbiol* 5(1) 25-31 (2002)

[31] Rödel R, Freyer A, Bittner T, Schäfer V, Hunfeld KP. In vitro activities of faropenem, ertapenem, imipenem and meropenem against Borrelia burgdorferi s.l. *Int J Antimicrob Agents.* 30(1):83-6. (2007)

[32] Freidank HM, Losch P, Vögele H et al. In Vitro Susceptibilities of Chlamydia pneumoniae Isolates from German Patients and Synergistic Activity of Antibiotic Combinations. *Antimicrobial Agents and Chemotherapy*, 43(7) 1808-1810, (1999)

[33] Cimmino MA, Accardo S. Long term treatment of chronic Lyme arthritis with benzathine penicillin. *Ann Rheum Dis.* 51(8):1007-8 (1992).

[34] Dever LL, Jorgensen JH, Barbour AG. In vitro activity of vancomycin against the spirochete Borrelia burgdorferi. *Antimicrob Agents Chemother.* 37(5):1115-21 (1993).

[35] Stricker RB. Counterpoint: long-term antibiotic therapy improves persistent symptoms associated with lyme disease. *Clin Infect Dis.* 45(2), 149-57 (2007).

[36] Ziska MH, Donta ST, Demarest FC, Physician preferences in the diagnosis and treatment of Lyme disease in the Unites States. *Infection* 24(2) 182-186 (1996)

[37] Maloy AL, Black RD, Segurola RJ Jr. Lyme disease complicated by the Jarisch-Herxheimer reaction. *J Emerg Med.* 16(3):437-8. (1998).

[38] Ljøstad U, Skogvoll E, Eikeland R et al. Oral doxycycline versus intravenous ceftriaxone for European Lyme neuroborreliosis: a multicentre, non-inferiority, double-blind, randomised trial. *Lancet Neurol.* 7(8):690-5. (2008) Erratum in: *Lancet Neurol.* 7(8):675 (2008).

[38] Bonnet JP, Abid L, Dabhar A, Lévy A, Soulier Y, Blangy S. Early biliary pseudolithiasis during ceftriaxone therapy for acute pyelonephritis in children: a prospective study in 34 children. *Eur J Pediatr Surg.* 10(6):368-71 (2000).

[39] Webster GF, Graber EM. Antibiotic treatment for acne vulgaris. *Semin Cutan Med Surg.* 27(3):183-7 (2008).

[40] Leiva M, Ruiz-Bravo A, Jimenez-Valera M. Effects of telithromycin in in vitro and in vivo models of lipopolysaccharide-induced airway inflammation. *Chest.* 134(1):20-9 (2008).

[41] Klempner MS, Hu LT, Evans J et al. Two controlled trials of antibiotic treatment in patients with persistent symptoms and a history of Lyme disease. *N Engl J Med.* 345(2):85-92 (2001).

[42] Hodzic E, Feng S, Holden K, Freet KJ, Barthold SW. Persistence of Borrelia burgdorferi following antibiotic treatment in mice. *Antimicrob Agents Chemother.* 52(5):1728-36 (2008).

[43] Yrjänäinen H, Hytönen J, Song XY, Oksi J, Hartiala K, Viljanen MK. Anti-tumor necrosis factor-alpha treatment activates Borrelia burgdorferi spirochetes 4 weeks after ceftriaxone treatment in C3H/He mice. *J Infect Dis.* 195(10):1489-96 (2007).

[44] Bennet L, Stjernberg L, Berglund J. Effect of gender on clinical and epidemiologic features of Lyme borreliosis. *Vector Borne Zoonotic Dis.* 7(1):34-41 (2007).

[45] Jarefors S, Bennet L, You E et al. Lyme borreliosis reinfection: might it be explained by a gender difference in immune response? *Immunology* 118(2):224-32 (2006).

[46] Cameron DJ. Generalizability in two clinical trials of Lyme disease. *Epidemiol Perspect Innov.* 17;3:12 (2006).

[47] Bransfield R, Brand S, Sherr V. Treatment of patients with persistent symptoms and a history of Lyme disease. *N Engl J Med.* 345(19):1424-5 (2001)

[48] Donta ST Treatment of patients with persistent symptoms and a history of Lyme disease. *N Engl J Med.* 8;345(19):1424 (2001)

[49] Cairns V, Godwin J. Post-Lyme borreliosis syndrome: a meta-analysis of reported symptoms. *Int J Epidemiol.* 34(6):1340-5. (2005).

[50] 22. Auwaerter PG. Point: Antibiotic Therapy Is Not the Answer for Patients with Persisting Symptoms Attributable to Lyme Disease. *Clinical Infectious Diseases.* 45:2, 143-148 (2007)

[51] Bakken JS, Dumler S. Human granulocytic anaplasmosis. *Infect Dis Clin North Am.* 22(3):433-48 (2008).

[52] Swanson SJ, Neitzel D, Reed KD, Belongia EA. Coinfections acquired from ixodes ticks. *Clin Microbiol Rev.* 19(4):708-27 (2006).

[53] Corapi KM, Gupta S, Liang MH. Management of Lyme disease. *Expert Rev Anti Infect Ther.* 6(2):241-50 (2008).

No financial conflicts. 2011-02-06. The contribution cannot replace a visit to the doctor. The authors distance themselves expressly from all contents of linked external Internet pages and do not endorse such content. This text was prepared with great care. However, no liability whatever can be accepted for its accuracy, especially in relation to dosages by the authors.